A WHOLE LIFE NOURISHED

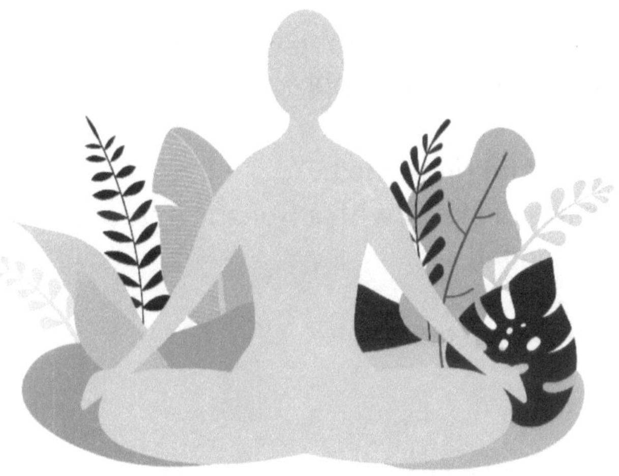

Plant-Based Living with a Holistic Approach

Diane Randall, M.A., CHC

A Whole Life Nourished:
Plant-Based Living with a Holistic Approach
Diane Randall

ISBN 979-8-218-39794-4

Published by:

Diane Randall, M.A., CHC

diane@dianerandallconsults.com

Table of Contents

Dedication

To my dearest Miles, Malcolm, and all the grandchildren I have yet to meet.

As I began writing this book, I couldn't help but think of each of you and the future that lies ahead.

My purpose in writing it is not simply to impart knowledge, but also to leave a legacy of love and dedication for a better world—one that is healthy, joyful, and environmentally conscious.

My greatest desire is for you to inherit a thriving planet filled with abundance and boundless opportunities.

As you continue to grow and discover new things in the world, always remember that your choices have the potential to create change. Whether it's opting for plant-based meals, taking care of the environment, or spreading kindness wherever you go, never forget that you have the power to make a positive impact on the world around you.

With all my love and optimism for the future.

Acknowledgments

It's hard to put into words how thankful I am for all the people who helped make *A Whole Life Nourished: Plant-Based Living with a Holistic Approach* a reality. There are no words that can truly express my gratitude.

I want to give a huge thank you to all the incredible listeners of the Plant-Based Curious Podcast. Your curiosity and enthusiasm for exploring the world of plant-based living have been the main inspiration throughout this experience. Your encouragement means everything to me.

I would like to express my immense gratitude to all the wonderful teachers who have guided me in the areas of spiritual growth, holistic health, personal development, and nutrition. Your wisdom and support have continually inspired me, and I am deeply appreciative of the profound influence you have had on my life.

Last but certainly not least, I want to express my sincerest gratitude to you, dear reader. Your decision on this journey, and for that, I am immensely thankful. My ultimate aspiration is for the thoughts and revelations shared in these pages to ignite something inside of you and motivate you to lead your most fulfilling and nourished life.

I want to express my sincerest gratitude to all of you for joining me on this journey. Here's to a future filled with good health, joy, and abundance!

With heartfelt appreciation,
Diane Randall, M.A., CHC

Introduction

Welcome to *A Whole Life Nourished: Plant-Based Living with a Holistic Approach*. I'm Diane Randall, your partner on this transformative journey toward a healthier, happier, and more fulfilling lifestyle.

Are you ready to unlock the secrets to a life full of vitality, purpose, and joy? Join me as we explore the profound connection between your dietary choices, physical health, emotional balance, and spiritual growth. This book isn't simply a collection of information—think of this book as your roadmap for holistic living, a demonstration from my many years of experience as a wellness consultant, podcast host, and passionate advocate for plant-based lifestyles.

Picture a morning when you wake up feeling invigorated, fueled by nourishing meals that delight your senses and uplift your soul. This is the essence of plant-based living—a lifestyle that extends beyond mere sustenance to embrace every facet of your existence.

But let's rewind a bit. My journey began in St. Louis, Missouri, a city renowned for its robust culture and delicious food, as well as being the home to the iconic Gateway Arch. Growing up, I was accustomed to the traditional American diet, but it took a toll on my health from a young age. As a young adult, I struggled with hypertension, high cholesterol, and other health problems. I was a walking example of the dangers that came with the familiar yet destructive foods I consumed.

My journey toward better health was not without its struggles—there were misunderstandings, societal pressures, and the weight of expectations to overcome. However, through these challenges, I found the realization and motivation to transform my life and improve my well-being.

This book is a guide filled with strategies, tools, and insights that have transformed not only my own life but also the lives of many others. It covers everything from mastering plant-based cooking to cultivating purpose, mindfulness, and self-reflection. Each chapter is a valuable resource of knowledge and skills intended to empower you on your journey toward successfully embracing a plant-based lifestyle.

But here's the thing: plant-based living isn't only about what you eat. It's about nourishing your entire being—mind, body, and spirit. It's about cultivating a lifestyle that honors your health, respects the planet, and fosters a profound sense of connection to yourself and the world around you.

As we journey together, my goal is to create a space for learning, growth, and mutual support. This isn't simply a book—it's a community, united by a shared commitment to wellness and compassion. Whether you're a seasoned plant-based enthusiast or a curious newcomer, there's something here for everyone. Let's inspire and uplift each other as we embark on this incredible adventure toward a whole life nourished.

Are you ready to embrace the transformative power of plant-based living? Let's dive in and discover the extraordinary possibilities that await us on this journey toward holistic wellness.

CHAPTER 1

My Transition to Plant-Based Living

Imagine this as the opening scene of a movie, where the adventure is about to begin in full force. In this chapter, I'll share my personal and reflective experiences from my past, including health challenges, and how my perspectives evolved to ultimately inspire some life-changing choices.

In this chapter, I will:

- Share my upbringing in St. Louis, Missouri, a place not typically associated with plant-based living.

- Recount how witnessing the slaughter of a chicken as a child impacted my views on animals and food.

- Reveal the health challenges I faced, including high blood pressure, cholesterol problems, and digestive issues.

- Outline the first steps I took toward adopting a plant-based diet.

- Present how I transitioned to a plant-based diet via the gradual evolution of my eating habits.

My adventure begins in St. Louis, Missouri, nestled in the heart of the Midwest—home of the iconic arch and delicious BBQ. Back in the day, animals were not a common sight in my everyday life; it was mostly limited to trips to the zoo or occasional visits to nearby farms. These experiences felt distant and did not provide a thorough understanding of the animal kingdom.

Everything changed one fateful day when I was nine years old on my great-grandparents' Mississippi farm. That was the day I saw a chicken get killed, and let me say, this experience made my nine-year-old self think. Witnessing that moment had a profound effect on me. It completely changed my perspective on where our food comes from and how animals are treated in the process. It was a pivotal event in my life, shaping my views on animals and their sentience.

Despite this, it took a long time for me to truly understand my relationship with animals and see them as more than food sources.

Once adulthood descended upon me, I was caught off guard. My once unbreakable sense of invincibility was shattered as I began to face serious health problems. Monitoring my high blood pressure and cholesterol levels became a draining and unwelcome part of my daily routine. In addition, my persistent digestive issues left me feeling exhausted and drained. A preliminary diagnosis of Crohn's disease from an upper gastrointestinal endoscopy added to my worries, until further tests proved it wrong.

My doctor's stern warning about the increased chances of heart disease and stroke was a jarring wake-up call, compelling me to reassess my daily habits. This difficult experience led me to contemplate societal expectations surrounding nutrition and the true key to living a healthy life.

The switch to a plant-based diet was not an immediate transition for me. Instead, it was more of a gradual shift that took time to develop. It started with small changes, like giving up beef and sugary drinks. While this may seem insignificant, it was the spark that ignited the transformation in my eating habits and overall focus on health, so in a sense, it was the pivotal point in my life's story. This phase wasn't simply about cutting out certain foods; it also involved incorporating more fruits, vegetables, and whole grains into my diet, setting the foundation for a healthier lifestyle.

As my health steadily improved, my understanding and outlook on veganism evolved as well. Initially, it was solely about improving my physical health. But as I delved deeper into the ethical and environmental implications of consuming animal products, my perspective shifted. Veganism became more than a dietary choice; it became a lifestyle dedicated to reducing harm to animals and the planet we share. My empathy for animals grew as I learned more about their suffering, marking a pivotal moment in my journey. Animals were no longer mere sources of sustenance; they were living beings with their own inherent right to exist and experience happiness.

How we shift to a plant-based way of life is different for each of us. Some give up animal products overnight, while others remove them gradually over time. For many of us, cheese is often the last thing to go.

For most people, this journey is an emotional rollercoaster when the realities of animal agriculture are staring us in the face. Trust that, ultimately, you will be rewarded with improvements to your health and personal growth. You'll have a deep awareness of how your decisions affect not only yourself but also the world around you.

This journey serves as a powerful reminder of the interconnectedness of all things in life.

CHAPTER 2

Grasping the Basics of Plant-Based Nutrition

There's no doubt there are misconceptions around plant-based diets, with one of the most popular and widespread being that eating soy gives men breasts. This is simply not true.

A common mistake many people make when they become vegan is to rely on pre-made, processed foods. Going this route will not likely improve your health. With some basic tools under your belt, you can thrive on a plant-based lifestyle. Remember to choose mostly whole foods—foods that you probably already enjoy—and replace your protein sources with plant proteins. You don't have to eat tofu, but it's not a bad option and it's versatile as it takes on the flavors of sauces and marinades. Whether you're new to this lifestyle or fully dedicated, this chapter will serve as your guide to the nutritional aspects of living a plant-based life.

At the core of plant-based nutrition lies a simple principle: consuming foods derived from plants provides you with the nutrients you need for optimum health. Plants encompass an array of wholesome options such as fruits, vegetables, grains, nuts, seeds, and legumes. By prioritizing whole and minimally processed foods, you can tap into the inherent goodness of these ingredients while gradually reducing your intake of animal products. It's about embracing a well-rounded and nourishing diet that stems directly from the Earth. It's also about understanding your motivation for making this lifestyle shift.

The idea of switching to a plant-based diet may be intimidating, especially if you're used to eating a lot of meat. However, don't worry, I'm here to cover the fundamental aspects of plant-based nutrition and tackle any questions or worries you may have.

Let's address some misconceptions before we delve into the specifics of plant-based nutrition.

These myths often circulate around this dietary approach and it's important to clarify them.

Myth 1: Plant-Based Diets Don't Provide Enough Nutrients

Despite this common misconception, plant-based diets are abundant in essential nutrients.

A concern among many, and likely a question most vegans have been asked at one time or another is: Where do you get your protein? Here's the truth—protein is not only found in meat. Plants have your back when it comes to protein. Think legumes, tofu, and quinoa, which are the plant world's muscle builders. You can get enough protein and enjoy a variety of delicious meals with a plant-based diet.

Leafy greens such as kale, spinach, and collard greens are rich sources of iron, calcium, and vitamin K; nuts and seeds like almonds, walnuts, chia seeds, and flaxseeds provide healthy fats and essential nutrients.

Whole grains such as quinoa, brown rice, and oats provide a mix of protein, fiber, and complex carbohydrates. Fruits and vegetables like berries, citrus fruits, broccoli, and sweet potatoes are packed with vitamins and antioxidants that benefit overall health.

Iron and calcium are found in spinach, lentils, and chickpeas. For calcium specifically, there's no need to look further than fortified plant milks, almonds, beans, lentils and leafy greens.

While it's true that vitamin B12 is mainly found in animal products, there's an easy solution: fortified foods and supplements. It's like giving your diet a little high-five with an extra boost.

The takeaway here is that a well-planned vegan diet isn't solely about cutting things out; it's about variety and balance. By including a rainbow of plant foods in your meals, you're not only covering all your nutritional bases but also enjoying a diverse and tasty diet. The next time someone asks about nutrients and veganism, you can tell them it's about smart choices and delicious variety.

Take Action: Plan Meals with Nutrient-Rich Foods

To ensure your body receives all the essential nutrients, incorporate a diverse range of these nutrient-rich foods into your diet. For instance, try a spinach salad topped with chickpeas and paired with an almond dressing. Not only will you savor a burst of delicious flavors, but you'll also benefit from a good source of iron, protein, and healthy fats.

Myth 2: Plant-Based Diets Are Expensive

Another myth about veganism is that it's expensive. You might think going vegan means you have to buy hard-to-find specialty products. Many people start their vegan journeys purchasing meat substitutes and vegan cheeses—cheese being the number one thing most vegans miss. However, relying on processed and packaged foods is not the optimum path to health or the best option for your wallet.

Plant-based eating can be more budget-friendly than diets heavy in animal products. For example, beans and legumes are highly nutritious and versatile, far less expensive than beef and pork, and you won't need to drain the fat before assembling your dish. Whole grains like brown rice and quinoa are not only affordable but they are also packed with nutrients you won't find in chicken. Additionally, tofu and tempeh are nutritious alternatives to animal proteins and can substitute for eggs in a tofu scramble and tofu eggless salad, or chicken when marinated and added to stir-fries, roasted vegetables, stews, and casseroles.

The key to a budget-friendly vegan diet is to stick to whole foods. As mentioned in Myth 1 above, we're talking beans, grains, veggies, fruits—nature's original fast food. These items are often cheaper than meat and processed foods, especially if you buy them in bulk. Imagine whipping up a hearty bean chili or a veggie stir-fry. Not only are these meals kind to your wallet, but they're also super nutritious and delicious.

Sure, there are plenty of fancy vegan products out there, but these are more like the cherry on top, not the whole sundae. You don't need them to have a satisfying vegan diet. Think of them as occasional treats or convenience options, rather than everyday necessities.

Another tip? Shop seasonal and local whenever possible. Seasonal produce is often less expensive and fresher, and shopping locally supports farmers in your area, which is always a nice bonus.

Being vegan doesn't mean you have to spend a fortune. With some smart shopping and a focus on whole, plant foods, you can eat well, save money, and enjoy a variety of delicious meals. It's like having your vegan cake and eating it too—cost-effective and conscientious!

Take Action: Creative Ways to Stay on Budget

To stay on budget while following a plant-based diet, try meal planning, buying in bulk, cooking at home, shopping for sales, and making healthy snacks rather than purchasing pre-packaged ones.

Myth 3: Plant-Based Diets Are Bland and Tasteless

One of the greatest joys of adopting a plant-based diet is discovering the diverse and delicious flavors it offers. There's no need to compromise on taste for the sake of health. Get creative with spices like cumin, coriander, and turmeric to add depth to your dishes. Expand your palate by exploring different cuisines such as Indian and Mediterranean, which offer alternative plant ingredients and cultural traditions. Don't be afraid to be adventurous with your cooking and incorporate ingredients like tofu, tempeh, and seitan for added flavor and texture.

Take Action: Spice Up Your Meals

To add some excitement to your meals, get creative in the kitchen! Use a variety of spices and herbs to elevate your dishes. For instance, try adding cumin, coriander, and paprika to your chickpea stew for a delicious Moroccan-inspired flavor. Not only will these spices enhance the taste of your dish, but they also offer antioxidant benefits.

Myth 4: Switching to a Plant-Based Diet Is Challenging

Adopting a plant-based lifestyle can be made easier with the right approaches. There are no shortages of resources available in the vegan space, and much of it is free. Follow vegan influencers on social media—YouTube and Instagram are two of the best platforms where plant-based people share content. Once you find a few you like, visit their websites for recipes, and sign up for their email lists for new creations to be delivered right to your inbox.

For eating on-the-go or at a restaurant, here are some useful suggestions:

Take Action: Plant-Based Options for On-the-Go and Dining Out

- Avoid the hassle of finding plant-based options while out by packing your own snacks, such as nuts, fruits, and energy bars.

- Plan ahead and research restaurants to discover those that have plant-based menu items. Many places now have dedicated menus or clearly designate plant-based dishes.

- When traveling, choose accommodations with kitchen facilities so you can easily prepare your own meals.

- Look for restaurants that have vegan or plant-based menu items; they often have creative and delicious plant-based choices.

- Don't be afraid to ask for substitutions or modifications to your order when dining out. Most restaurants are accommodating and willing to help you stick to your plant-based goals.

Myth 5: Plant-Based Diets Are Only for Vegans and Vegetarians

Plant-based diets are quite versatile and accommodating, and they are inclusive and adaptable. While some people who follow plant-based diets may also identify as vegan or vegetarian, others choose this path for reasons related to their health, ethics, or the environment. It is not limited to one specific group of individuals.

Take Action: Be Flexible

Don't be afraid to tailor your plant-based diet to fit your personal preferences and needs. Start by adding more plant-based meals to your current eating habits, and gradually decrease your intake of animal products. This gradual shift can make the transition smoother and easier to maintain in the long run.

Myth 6: Plant-Based Diets Don't Supply Adequate Protein

The infamous misconception about protein! It's often assumed that animal products are the only sources of protein. However, by including a diverse range of plant proteins such as leafy greens, beans, lentils, tofu, nuts, and seeds in your diet, you can easily fulfill your daily protein needs.

Take Action: Incorporate a Variety of Protein Sources

Don't limit yourself to beans and lentils; try different options like tofu, tempeh, seitan, and plant-based protein powders. Mix things up and keep your meals interesting and nutrient-rich. For instance, a quinoa and black bean salad is an excellent choice for a protein-packed and tasty meal.

Myth 7: Plant-Based Diets Are Too Restrictive

Some people may have concerns that a plant-based diet is too restrictive. However, with the wide variety of fruits, vegetables, grains, legumes, nuts, and seeds readily available now, there are countless options to choose from.

Take Action: Discover and Innovate

Immerse yourself in the realm of plant-based cuisine. Test new dishes, ingredients, and cultural flavors. Wander through your nearby farmers' market to uncover fresh, seasonal produce and novel types of fruits and veggies, such as lion's mane or oyster mushrooms and jackfruit. Let your curiosity guide you in the kitchen, and you'll unlock a world of possibilities with plant-based foods. For example, try a quinoa and vegetable stir-fry for a tasty and nourishing meal that highlights the adaptability of plant-based ingredients.

Essential Nutrients to Include in a Plant-Based Diet

Let's now discuss important nutrients to keep in mind when following a plant-based diet.

- Protein: Necessary for overall health, you can find it in legumes (such as lentils, chickpeas, and beans), tofu, tempeh, nuts, and seeds.

- Iron: Great sources include lentils, chickpeas, beans, tofu, pumpkin seeds, quinoa, and fortified cereals.

- Calcium: You can get your calcium intake from fortified plant milks, leafy green vegetables (like kale and Bok choy), almonds, tahini, and fortified tofu.

- Omega-3 Fatty Acids: These are abundant in flaxseeds, chia seeds, hemp seeds, walnuts, and supplements made from algae.

- Vitamin B12: Vital for vegans, it can be found in fortified plant-based milks, nutritional yeast, and supplements.

- Vitamin D: You can obtain it through sunlight exposure, fortified foods, or supplements.

Take Action: Strive for Balance

As you transition to a plant-based diet, it's important to monitor your nutrient intake for optimal health. Here are some tips:

- Gradually incorporate more plant-based meals into your diet while decreasing animal products.

- Include a variety of food groups in your meals to ensure you get all the essential nutrients.

- Experiment with new plant-based recipes and find creative ways to substitute traditional ingredients.

- Educate yourself about the principles of plant-based nutrition so you can make informed choices about your diet.

- Be mindful of how different foods affect your overall well-being. For example, consuming vitamin D-fortified plant-based milk can help maintain healthy levels of this essential nutrient.

Throughout this chapter, I have dispelled common misconceptions, offered helpful advice, and equipped you with the necessary information to embark on a successful plant-based journey. It's not solely about your food choices, but also about fully embracing this nourishing way of life. Keep an open mind, stay motivated, and let's continue this wonderful journey together.

CHAPTER 3

The Holistic Connection

Plant-based nutrition has a powerful influence on your overall wellness. If you haven't yet experienced this for yourself, this chapter delves into how this lifestyle impacts your mental and spiritual wellness, in addition to your physical well-being.

Let's start our discussion with the concept of mindful eating. In essence, it involves being completely aware and in the present while consuming your meals. This includes truly appreciating each bite, utilizing all your senses, and acknowledging the underlying emotions behind your food choices. But why is this important, and how can it positively impact you?

The practice of mindful eating goes beyond being a fad—it has the power to transform your relationship with food. By slowing down and paying attention to sensations and experiences while eating, you can improve digestion, develop healthier eating habits, and gain a new level of gratitude for the nourishment your body receives.

Simply put, it's not simply about *what* you eat but *how* you eat that makes a difference.

Beginning Your Mindful Eating Journey

We have become a society of the easily distracted, to our detriment. Practicing mindfulness as you begin your plant-based journey will help remind you of all the reasons this journey will benefit you, the animals, and the planet.

Take Action Tip 1:

Here are some easy steps to get you started with mindful eating:

- Eliminate distractions during meals, which could mean turning off the TV and putting away your phone.

- Pay attention to your senses; take time to appreciate the textures, flavors, and smells of your food.

- Listen to your body's signals and recognize when you're hungry and when you're comfortably satisfied to avoid overeating.

- Practice gratitude by taking a moment to be thankful for the food on your plate—the Earth that provides it and the hands that nurtured and cultivated it.

Incorporating Mindful Eating into Daily Life

Making mindful eating a part of your daily routine will help you create healthy habits and avoid slippery slopes that could derail your efforts. Incorporate some or all of the following suggestions to help you do that.

Take Action Tip 2: Choosing Food with Mindfulness

Here are some easy steps to get you started with mindful eating:

- Plan your meals in advance, considering both taste and nutrition. For example, look forward to a healthy breakfast by preparing overnight oats in the evening. Top it with fruit, nuts, or seeds in the morning and enjoy!

- Choose whole, unprocessed foods while grocery shopping. It's also a good idea to wash and cut vegetables ahead of time so that meal prep is a breeze, and snacks are handy.

- Be mindful of portion sizes to prevent overeating. Many of us tend to put more on our plates than what we can eat. Start smaller than usual and know you can always go back for more if you're still hungry.

- Get creative in the kitchen; try new recipes and experiment with herbs and spices. Also, don't be afraid of trying vegetables or other ingredients that may be new to you. A new world is opening.

- Savor each bite. This is the embodiment of mindfulness. If you tend to eat fast, slow down, which also helps with the digestion process.

- As you're preparing your meals, remind yourself of the positive impact on the environment and think about how your food choices affect the world around you.

Establishing the Right Atmosphere

The environment you are in can greatly impact your eating habits, therefore it is important to understand how to create an ideal setting for mindful eating.

Take Action Tip 3: Creating an Environment for Mindful Eating

Here are some tips on how to design a space that promotes mindful eating:

- Choose a peaceful, distraction-free spot to savor your meals. For example, if your kitchen is a busy spot with family members eating at different times, enjoy your meals in the dining room, even if you typically only use it during holidays and with guests.

- Utilize warm and inviting lighting and decor to establish a calming ambiance. Consider lighting a candle. Use stemware or a fancy glass for your water, instead of drinking from a water bottle.

- Break the habit of eating while multitasking or watching screens. This can be achieved by designating a specific area for dining and leaving your phone in another room.

- To inspire a mindful mindset before sitting down to eat, consider uplifting conversations with loved ones as you're preparing the meal, or reading or listening to motivational messages. They help contribute to a mindful mindset.

Remaining Present During Social Meals and Restaurant Outings

Eating with others can be difficult for maintaining mindfulness, especially if you are the only one following a plant-based diet. Let's work through this together.

Take Action Tip 4: Practicing Mindful Eating with Others

Here are some tips for staying mindful during social meals and dining out:

- Set your intention before the meal; make a conscious decision to stay present and make mindful choices.

- Focus on the connections and conversations with those around you.

- Consider sharing dishes as a way to be mindful of portion sizes and to entice omnivores with the delicious flavors of a plant-based dish.

- If you want to remain mindful of moderation, consider sharing a dessert and fully enjoy every bite.

- Take a moment to express gratitude for the experience and the food provided.

Exploring the Effects of Diet on Mental and Emotional Health

From the benefits of omega-3 fatty acids and antioxidants to the fascinating gut-brain connection, your diet can play a significant role in your overall mental health.

Take Action Tip 5: Taking Care of Your Mind and Emotions

Here's how to nourish your mind and emotions through your food choices:

- Incorporate plant-based sources of omega-3s, such as flaxseeds, chia seeds, and walnuts.

- Indulge in the benefits of antioxidants found in berries, leafy greens, and nuts.

- Choose foods rich in fiber from plant sources for a happy and healthy gut microbiome. These include sweet potatoes, black beans, split peas, and almonds.

- Many plant foods contain the phytochemical quercetin, which can increase neurotransmitters like serotonin and dopamine in the brain and work to improve your mood. This phytochemical can be found in apples, berries, grapes, and kale, to name a few. There may be some truth to the proverb "An apple a day keeps the doctor away."

- Many foods from the standard American diet are known to cause inflammation, for example, refined carbs, sugary soft drinks, fried foods, and red meat. Chronic inflammation can lead to diseases such as diabetes, Alzheimer's, cancer, and heart disease. A diet with plenty of plant foods such as leafy greens, berries, nuts, and tomatoes with natural antioxidants and polyphenols has been shown to reduce inflammation in the body.

Finding Balance between the Physical, Mental, and Spiritual Elements of Life

Now, let's discuss the importance of balance because I'm talking about something bigger than what you put on your plate. It's about nourishing your physical, mental, and spiritual well-being for a truly satisfying life.

Take Action Tip 6 for Balance: Practical Strategies

Here are some practical strategies that can help you achieve balance. Incorporate these strategies into your daily routine for a well-rounded sense of wellness:

- Variety is the spice of life. Consider physical activity such as yoga, aerobics, strength training, swimming, cycling, walking, and Zumba, to name a few. If you haven't already, try Tabata, HIIT, spin, step, or Nia. By mixing up your routine, you won't get bored and your body's fitness won't plateau.

- Don't neglect rest, relaxation, quality sleep, and time away from all devices; these are essential for mental well-being.

- Practice mindfulness techniques like meditation and deep breathing to sharpen your mind.

- Explore your spiritual side by connecting with nature, journaling, praying, or having a gratitude practice.

This chapter highlights the idea that adopting a plant-based lifestyle is not only about what you consume, but rather a transformative journey that encompasses all aspects of your being. It encourages a reevaluation of one's relationship with food and its impact on self-discovery, personal growth, and overall holistic well-being.

By exploring mindful eating, understanding the link between nutrition and psychology, and incorporating physical, mental, and spiritual practices, you are on your way toward a nourishing way of life. Remember, it's not solely about the foods you eat, but also how you embrace this lifestyle in every aspect of your life.

Let's continue this journey together, nurturing our bodies, minds, and spirits. Our well-being deserves nothing less than our utmost care and attention.

CHAPTER 4

Nurturing Sustainable Practices

Now we will explore the world of sustainable living through plant-based practices—a thrilling adventure that not only enhances our physical and mental health but also positively impacts our planet. Throughout this chapter, we will examine the environmental effects of our eating habits, stress the importance of sustainable farming, and offer practical steps toward an eco-friendlier lifestyle.

The relationship between personal health and environmental impact is an essential one to consider. By being conscious of our food choices, we can make a positive impact on the world around us. Opting for a plant-based diet not only benefits our own well-being but also serves as a powerful means of combating climate change. It's a win-win situation for us and the Earth.

Why it's important:

- Animal agriculture is a major contributor to greenhouse gas emissions. By choosing plant-based foods, you can significantly reduce your carbon footprint.

- Meat production requires a significant amount of water. In contrast, plant-based diets are more sustainable for our water resources.

- Opting for plants instead of meat helps protect biodiversity by decreasing deforestation and protecting habitats.

Sarah's Journey to a Greener Lifestyle

Introducing Sarah, an avid nature enthusiast who made the conscious decision to switch to a plant-based diet. Prior to this change, she regularly consumed meat as part of her meals. However, after switching to a plant-based diet, she did some calculations and was amazed to see how much less she was contributing to greenhouse gas emissions. Not only did this make her feel better about her impact on the environment, but she also experienced improvements in her health and overall well-being.

The relationship between sustainable agriculture and a plant-based lifestyle is crucial to understand. Traditional farming methods can have negative impacts, but by adopting sustainable practices, we can benefit both ourselves and the environment. As conscious consumers, we have the power to support sustainable farming and make a positive impact on the world. Let's explore this connection further.

Drawbacks of Traditional Agriculture:

- Conventional farming practices can harm the soil and contaminate water with harmful chemicals, causing damage to human lives and the planet.

- As mentioned, raising animals for meat contributes significantly to greenhouse gas emissions, and it's also a factor in deforestation. These animal agriculture practices take a toll on Earth's health.

Advantages of Sustainable Farming:

- Sustainable agriculture techniques prioritize maintaining healthy soil through methods such as crop rotation and composting. This results in healthier crops and reduced use of chemicals.

- Organic farming eliminates the use of synthetic pesticides and GMOs, benefiting both consumers and farmers. Veganic farming takes this a step further by avoiding using fertilizers that contain animal byproducts.

- Supporting small-scale organic farms that produce locally also reduces the environmental impact of food transportation and supports local communities.

The Transformation of David's Farm

David, a farmer from a rural area, made the courageous decision to transition from traditional farming methods to sustainable and organic practices. As a result, he witnessed a significant change—the health of his soil improved drastically, and local wildlife flourished. His farm quickly became a model for sustainable agriculture in the community, inspiring others to follow in his footsteps and embrace eco-friendly practices.

Becoming Familiar with Eco-Friendly Food Certifications

Knowing the meaning behind food certifications and labels can be key to making responsible decisions about what you consume. Certifications such as USDA Organic, Fairtrade Certified, and Rainforest Alliance Certified guarantee that the products you select adhere to strict environmental and social guidelines.

Supporting Sustainable Agriculture through Plant-Based Choices

When you choose a plant-based lifestyle, you're essentially saying no to resource-intensive animal products. And guess what? You're also saying yes to supporting eco-friendly practices.

Mia's Environmentally Conscious Shopping

Mia made a promise to only purchase products that had eco-friendly certifications. She soon discovered that numerous plant-based options proudly displayed these certifications, which resulted in her decision-making process being effortless and free of guilt. Knowing that her daily meals were contributing to a better world made her heart smile.

Moving Beyond Food

Adopting a seasonal diet and incorporating more fruits and vegetables is not only beneficial for your health, but it also helps reduce the energy required for storage and transportation. And that's a win for our planet!

Here are some easy steps to lead an eco-friendlier lifestyle:

- Start with making small adjustments in your daily routine, such as composting, recycling, and replacing single-use plastics with reusable alternatives. For example, say goodbye to disposable water bottles and switch to a stylish reusable one, and make or purchase reusable produce bags for shopping.

- Conserve valuable resources like energy and water by using energy-efficient appliances and being mindful of water usage. You can even install efficient low-flow showerheads to decrease water consumption.

Alex's Commitment to a Sustainable Lifestyle

Alex made the decision to fully embrace an eco-friendly lifestyle, going beyond his dietary choices. He drastically cut down on waste, became skilled in composting, and installed solar panels on his roof. Not only did he decrease his impact on the environment, but he also inspired his neighbors to join the green movement.

In Chapter 4, you learned how your decisions can have a positive impact on the environment. By incorporating eco-friendly practices into your daily routine and embracing a plant-based diet, you are becoming an advocate for our planet. These real-life examples demonstrate that making sustainable choices isn't solely about saving Earth; it's also about personal fulfillment and inspiring others to do the same. It's a call to action, motivating you to move toward a more sustainable future. Through conscious choices in your eating habits and lifestyle, you can make a significant difference, not only for yourself but for the entire world around you.

CHAPTER 5

Tips for Incorporating a Plant-Based Diet into Your Busy Life

This chapter will guide you in seamlessly integrating a plant-based diet into your hectic daily routine. I understand that life can be chaotic, but that doesn't mean you have to give up on your goal of eating more plant-based foods. In this chapter, I will address common challenges and equip you with useful strategies for meal planning, grocery shopping, and cooking. My goal is to demonstrate that not only is a plant-based diet achievable, but it can also bring joy to your everyday life.

Becoming an Expert in Meal Planning and Preparation

Transitioning to a plant-based lifestyle may seem overwhelming, particularly when it comes to meal planning and preparation. But don't worry, with the right approach, you can make this change seamless and stress-free. Let's discover some useful methods for saving time, staying on track, and achieving a well-rounded diet.

When life gets hectic, it can be tough to find time for meal planning. That's why it's important to set aside a specific time each week to focus on it. This could be a peaceful Sunday afternoon or another suitable day that works for you. Use this dedicated time to browse cookbooks or search online for recipe inspiration. Aim to create a menu with a variety of plant proteins, such as beans, lentils, tofu, tempeh, nuts, seeds, and whole grains like quinoa, brown rice, and whole wheat pasta. Don't forget to include plenty of fresh fruits and veggies—they are full of essential nutrients!

With a diverse menu, you'll never get bored of your plant-based diet. Tired of eating the same thing every day? Try branching out into different global cuisines, like Indian dishes made with dal, Middle Eastern falafel, Mexican bean burritos, or Thai curries. Get creative and experiment with new ingredients and flavors to keep mealtime interesting and enjoyable.

For mid-day energy slumps, the key is to opt for nutritious snacks that not only satisfy your cravings but also provide essential nutrients.

To spend less time in the kitchen, and to have ingredients at the ready when you are running short on time, consider the following tips:

- Batch wash and cut vegetables soon after your trip to the grocery store. Set aside time each week to do this and you will be grateful when you come home from work late and need to put a meal on the table quickly.

- Cook large portions of essential foods, such as grains, beans, and roasted vegetables, that you can use in several recipes for multiple meals throughout the week.

- Prepare hearty salads, savory soups, or comforting stews in advance to have quick and easy meal options at your fingertips.

- Choose meals that can be frozen and reheated, another useful strategy that is perfect for those hectic days when time is limited.

Essential Cooking Tips

Preparing a delicious meal doesn't have to be overwhelming. If you have a favorite dish, veganize it by replacing the meat with lentils, for example. Here are additional tips:

- Embrace simple yet healthy dishes such as stir-fries, wraps, and grain bowls.

- Save time with pre-cut vegetables—either vegetables you've cut yourself or purchased that way—and canned beans for faster cooking.

- Discover ways to enhance flavor with spices and herbs without spending too much time or effort. There is likely a world of sauces and condiments that you have yet to try. Experiment. Do some research if you're so inclined.

Grocery Shopping and Cooking Advice

Let's become savvy shoppers and efficient cooks.

Shop Wisely:

- Focus on purchasing whole, unprocessed foods.

- Ensure you always have nuts, seeds, grains, and legumes in your pantry.

- Explore diverse markets for distinct ingredients and spices to add a burst of flavor to your dishes.

- Support sustainable farming at local farmers' markets. Much like supporting local artisans, communities thrive when we buy from small local growers. Many practice organic farming, even if they aren't certified as such. You will enjoy fresh produce and contribute to a healthier planet at the same time. This is a win for you, a win for local farmers, and a win for the planet.

Master the Art of Plant-Based Cooking:

- Learn fundamental cooking skills such as sautéing, roasting, and steaming.

- Keep things exciting by regularly experimenting with new recipes in your plant-based diet.

- Google recipes for specific ingredients you need to use. For example, if you have a head of broccoli in your fridge, enter "vegan recipes using broccoli" in the search field and see what comes up.

Essential Kitchen Tools and Equipment to Invest In

Ensure your kitchen is equipped with the necessary tools. Some of these items can be expensive so if budget is a concern, make these investments over time.

- Quality knives are a must for any kitchen.

- A high-speed blender can whip up a delicious smoothie with frozen fruit, purée soups, and turn ingredients like sunflower seeds, lemon and garlic into delectable sauces.

- Food processors are great for slicing, dicing, and chopping, and help reduce your time prepping ingredients. Great to have available if you batch wash and cut your vegetables.

- Consider appliances like slow cookers or Instant Pots for convenient meal preparation.

Striking a Balance Between a Busy Life and Healthy Nutrition

I understand—life can be chaotic, so here are some time-saving tips:

- Consider using meal delivery services or pre-made plant-based meal kits for convenience.

- Prepare parts of the dish in advance to save time, for example, make dressings and sauces during the time of the week you've set aside for meal planning.

Strategies for Eating Out and Attending Social Events

Don't let social gatherings hinder your plant-based journey:

- Do some research on restaurants beforehand to uncover plant-based menu items.

- Don't hesitate to ask for vegan alternatives while dining out.

- Bring a plant-based dish to potlucks or get-togethers, which can spark interesting conversations.

As a final point, it's important to remember that life can be unpredictable, and it's okay to be open-minded about your plant-based diet. I'm confident the practical methods and tips I've shared in this chapter will help you seamlessly incorporate a plant-based diet into your busy life. My ultimate goal is to make healthy, plant-based eating not only manageable but also enjoyable. By implementing these adaptable and realistic approaches, you will not only enhance your health but also contribute to environmental sustainability. With some careful planning and a touch of imagination, adopting a plant-based diet can become an enriching and essential component of your lifestyle. So go ahead and embrace the green goodness!

CHAPTER 6

Looking Beyond the Food on Your Plate – A Holistic Perspective on Veganism

Now is the time to widen our lens and take a good, hard look at veganism, and trust me, it's about so much more than salads and smoothies. It's a journey into a world where our choices ripple out to touch lives, the environment, and our sense of compassion.

Let's start by exploring the ethical heartbeat of veganism. Imagine every meal as a statement of kindness—where choosing plant-based options is like saying 'no thanks' to animal cruelty. It's not only about what we eat; it's about being mindful of the lives affected by our choices.

But hold on, there's an even bigger picture. Veganism and our planet—they're like best friends. This chapter will show you how eating plants is great for your health and I'll demonstrate why it's a high-five to Mother Earth. From shrinking your carbon footprint to giving a nod to water conservation, it's like giving the planet a little thank-you note with every meal.

Now, let's bust some myths. Heard the one about vegans not getting enough protein? Or that veganism is way too expensive? Spoiler alert: they're myths, and we'll dismantle them with facts and clarity. You'll see how veganism can be both nourishing and budget-friendly.

In addition to what's on your plate, veganism can kick-start a whole wave of positive changes. It's about community, about healthier lifestyles, and even about influencing economic choices toward more sustainable practices.

In this chapter, we're talking about a life choice that's brimming with empathy, responsibility, and care for our planet. By the end of this chapter, you'll see veganism in a whole new light—not solely as a dietary choice but as a path to a more compassionate, sustainable, and connected life. Ready to dive in? Let's get started and unfold the many layers of veganism together!

Understanding the Moral Ideals of Veganism

Let's dive into the heart of veganism, especially the part about animal rights. It's like opening a book on empathy and extending that empathy to every creature, big or small.

Think of veganism as more than a diet; it's a stand for compassion. At its core, veganism is about believing that every living being deserves respect and kindness—that they are not reserved for humans only. This perspective shifts how we view animals—not as commodities or resources, but as beings with their own rights and feelings.

This is where veganism shines. It's about extending a hand of moral consideration to all beings, whether they're a cow in the pasture, a sheep in the fields, or a rabbit in the wild. It's acknowledging that every animal has the right to live a life free from harm and exploitation.

Embracing veganism means saying 'no' to using animals for our gains. Again, this isn't limited to food—it encompasses everything from the leather in shoes to the entertainment in circuses. It's a commitment to finding alternatives that don't involve animal use or suffering.

When you look at it this way, veganism is more than a personal choice; it's a stance against the commodification of animal life. It's about recognizing that animals are here with us, not for us, and adjusting our choices to reflect that understanding. In doing so, we open to a world where compassion extends to every corner of our lives.

Species Equality

Now, let's talk about something interesting in veganism—the idea of species equality. It's a bit of a mind-bender but stick with me. Veganism throws a question into the ring: why do we consider humans to be above other animals? It's like looking at the world through a different lens, one that doesn't put humans at the center.

Veganism gets us thinking. It questions the long-held belief that humans are the top dogs (or, top species, if you will) on this planet. It's about challenging the notion that being human makes us inherently superior to other animals. Think about it: we all share the same Earth, breathe the same air, and live our lives. Veganism nudges us to consider a world where all species have their own intrinsic value.

This idea leads us to something called 'speciesism'—it's like racism or sexism but based on species. Veganism takes a stand against this. It says, "Hey, just because they're not human animals, it doesn't mean they deserve any less consideration or compassion." It's about recognizing that discrimination based on species has led us down a path where exploiting and mistreating animals has become too easy and too common.

When you start seeing things from a vegan perspective, it shifts the whole picture. It's not about humans versus other animals; it's about all of us sharing this planet. By embracing species equality, we open ourselves to a more equitable and compassionate world—one where every creature, regardless of its species, is treated with respect and kindness. It's a big step, but it's one that makes the journey of veganism all the more powerful and meaningful.

Sentience

This is a key part of the vegan puzzle—understanding that animals are sentient beings. It's a bit like realizing that the animals we share the planet with aren't simply moving around on autopilot. They feel things, just like us.

Here's the deal: animals can feel happiness, pain, hunger, fear, and a whole spectrum of emotions. It's fascinating, isn't it? When you watch a dog wagging its tail in excitement or a cat purring contentedly, it's clear they're feeling something. But it goes beyond our pets. Cows, pigs, chickens, sheep, goats—they too experience emotions. They can form bonds and show affection, and they can feel distress and pain.

As vegans, this understanding translates into a strong call for compassion. If animals can suffer, then they deserve our kindness and respect, right? It's about recognizing that every creature with the capacity to feel pain should also have the right to avoid it. This belief in sentience pushes vegans to advocate for animal rights and to live in a way that minimizes harm to these sentient beings.

When you start to see animals as sentient creatures, it changes your perspective on a lot of things. You begin to see them as fellow beings sharing this journey of life with us. That's a powerful realization—one that fuels the vegan commitment to treat all animals with the compassion and respect they deserve. It's a view that enriches the lives of animals and our lives as well, bringing a deeper sense of connection and empathy to our world.

The Reality of Animal Agriculture

When we peel back the curtain on animal agriculture, especially factory farming, the view can be quite sobering. Let's take a closer look at this.

This side of animal agriculture is often hidden, but it's important to understand it. Picture this: vast numbers of animals are kept in places that are more like crowded warehouses than farms. Space is a luxury they don't have, and the conditions? Well, they're often far from sanitary.

Imagine living your entire life in a space so cramped you can barely move. That's the reality for many animals in factory farms. They're packed in tightly, with little room to roam or even turn around. Beyond the physical discomfort for the animals, these conditions can lead to serious health problems and an inability to behave in a way that is their nature.

Here's a hard truth—in factory farming, dollars trump animal welfare. It's all about producing as much as possible, as fast as possible, and as cheaply as possible. This drive for profit can lead to some horrific inhumane practices, like animals not being given proper veterinary care or being subjected to procedures without pain relief.

When we talk about veganism, it goes beyond making healthier food choices; it's also about being aware of and standing against these kinds of practices. Understanding the reality of factory farming is a big part of why many choose a vegan lifestyle. It's about saying no to a system that treats animals as commodities and saying yes to living compassionately.

Cruelty to Animals

Let's talk about a rather tough topic in the world of factory farming—the cruelty animals face. It's not the easiest thing to think about, but it's crucial for understanding why many people choose veganism.

In large-scale farms, animals often go through harsh treatment. For instance, they might be mutilated as a part of standard farming procedures—think docking tails and debeaking— and this is typically done without any pain relief. Imagine being in their place, experiencing such pain and fear, and not understanding why it's happening. It's heartbreaking.

Another aspect is how these animals are confined. They don't get to roam, graze, or even move much. They're kept in spaces so small that their natural behaviors are completely stifled. There's also the emotional pain of separation—like calves being taken away from their mothers. These practices, often standard in factory farming, ignore the emotional well-being of the animals entirely.

When we talk about cruelty to animals in factory farms, it includes physical pain and emotional suffering. These practices can be hard to come to terms with, and they're a big reason why many people choose veganism. Once you know—particularly if you've witnessed the cruelty via a documentary or an undercover video—it's difficult to ignore. Veganism is a way to stand against such cruelty and advocate for a world where animals are treated with the compassion and respect they deserve. Making this shift isn't only good for the animals; it often brings a sense of alignment and peace to our own lives, knowing we're part of a kinder, more ethical way of living.

Environmental Impact

You might be surprised to learn how much of a footprint our appetite for animal products has on Mother Earth. It's quite a story, so let's unpack it.

When we think about environmental degradation and climate change, cars and factories often come to mind. But animal farming is a major player too. It's the elephant in the room of environmental issues. The emissions from millions of cows, pigs, and chickens add up, and not in a good way. We're talking methane and nitrous oxide—gases that are more potent than carbon dioxide in terms of trapping heat in our atmosphere. And the total greenhouse gases from animal agriculture outdoes those from all the cars, trains, and planes combined. It's a bit mind-boggling!

Animal farming is also incredibly thirsty work. It takes a lot of water to raise animals, not to mention the water needed to grow their feed. In a world where water scarcity is a growing concern, this is a big deal. It's equivalent to filling a bathtub to the brim for a single hamburger. That's a lot of water!

There's also the issue of water pollution. The runoff from these farms, loaded with fertilizers and animal waste, can end up in rivers and oceans. It's a domino effect—one thing leads to another, and before you know it, we have a whole host of environmental problems.

Deforestation is another major consequence. Forests are being chopped down at an alarming rate to make room for grazing or to grow feed. It's not only about losing trees; it's about losing entire ecosystems that are crucial for the planet's health.

Plus, when those trees go, all the carbon they've been storing gets released, which is like adding fuel to the climate change fire.

The story doesn't end there. This large-scale clearing of land leads to the loss of habitats, impacting wildlife and biodiversity. We're talking about animals losing their homes and plants disappearing that hold untold medicinal values. This not only affects wildlife but also indigenous communities that rely on these ecosystems for their way of life.

Animal farming is resource-intensive. When we take a hard look at the environmental impact of animal farming, it's clear why so many people are turning to veganism. Those committed to this lifestyle are making choices that are kinder to our planet, and they are helping to preserve the world for future generations. I'll talk more about this later in this chapter.

In a nutshell, animal agriculture's impact on the environment is vast and varied, from the air we breathe to the water we drink, and the ecosystems we rely on. Reducing our consumption of animal products can be a powerful way to lessen our environmental footprint. We all need to do our part to help reduce the impact on our planet, and reducing or eliminating animal products is the single most effective way for individuals to do that. Every plant-based meal is a step toward a more sustainable and healthier planet.

Embracing a plant-based lifestyle is like casting a vote for a greener, cleaner earth. It's a way of saying, "Hey, I care about our planet, and I'm going to do my bit to protect it."

Reasons to Embrace a Vegan Lifestyle

Let's chat about one of the most heartfelt reasons people decide to go vegan: compassion toward animals. It's a big motivator and it's the heart and soul of veganism. When you choose to go vegan, you're saying no to a system that doesn't treat animals with the kindness and respect they deserve.

Every time you opt for a plant-based burger over a beef one, or choose almond milk instead of cow's milk, you're doing more than simply making a dietary choice. You become part of a bigger movement that's reducing the demand for animal-based products. It's casting a vote for a kinder world.

Think of it this way: the fewer animal products bought, the less the demand, and eventually, this will lead to fewer animals being bred into a life of abuse and ultimately killed in factory farms. That's significant. It's about chipping away at a system that relies on animal suffering and saying, "Hey, there's a better, kinder way to do this."

Choosing veganism for animal compassion is about aligning your actions with your heart. It's a powerful way to stand up for those who can't speak for themselves and to make choices that reflect a deep respect for all living beings. There's something amazing about knowing that your everyday choices are contributing to a more compassionate world.

Improved Personal Health

Let's switch gears and talk about how going vegan is also a big win for your health. Let's delve into this wholesome world of plant-based goodness.

You know how we're always hearing about eating more fruits, veggies, nuts, and whole grains? Well, that's pretty much the basis of a vegan diet. These foods are like nature's little treasure chests, packed with vitamins, minerals, and fiber. It's like fueling your body with the best stuff out there.

Switching to a plant-based diet can be like giving your body a health shield. Studies have shown that vegans often have a lower risk of some major health issues, such as heart disease, high blood pressure, type 2 diabetes, and even some cancers. Eating a variety of plant foods means you're giving your body an extra layer of protection against health issues.

Chronic illnesses are also a big concern these days. Eating whole plant foods can help keep these illnesses in check. It's about reducing the bad stuff (like cholesterol and saturated fats, which are often high in animal products) and upping the good stuff (like heart-healthy fiber and antioxidants). It's equivalent to turning your meals into a health-boosting potion.

Embracing a vegan lifestyle for personal health is like giving your body a big high-five. You're choosing foods that not only taste good but also are beneficial for your health. Plus, there's the bonus of feeling great, knowing that your food choices are helping you live your healthiest life.

Environmental Sustainability

Switching to a vegan lifestyle can be a game-changer for our wonderful, beautiful, and somewhat stressed planet. Embracing plant-based alternatives does make a difference.

Imagine the Earth as a friend who's carrying way too much stuff. Animal farming is a bit like adding an extra-heavy backpack to what they're already carrying. It's tough on resources like land, water, and energy. When you choose plant-based options, you are lightening that load in the backpack. Plants generally require fewer resources to grow than raising animals, so each plant-based meal is a step toward easing the burden on our planet.

You've probably heard about climate change, right? It's like the Earth is running a fever because of all the greenhouse gases we're adding to the atmosphere. Animal agriculture is a big contributor to those gases, especially methane, which cows are famous for producing. By going vegan, you're helping to cut down those emissions, joining the growing population of people who have eliminated animal products, which means fewer cows are bred for milk and beef production. It's a way for you to help turn down the dial on the Earth's thermostat, or at the very least, prevent it from warming further.

Here's the cool part—when you choose vegan, you're not simply making a solitary choice. Like throwing a pebble into a pond, the ripples spread and create a bigger impact. Fewer animal products mean less demand for factory farming, which means more room for natural habitats, more forests, and cleaner air and water. It's a win-win-win!

Choosing a vegan lifestyle for the sake of environmental sustainability helps you become a champion for our planet. Every plant-based meal is a small victory in the fight against environmental stress. And the best part? You're doing it by enjoying delicious, earth-friendly foods. How awesome is that?

The Benefits of Veganism

The bigger picture of what veganism can do for us and our planet is like turning over a new leaf, both for our health and the environment.

First, a vegan lifestyle is like a lightweight backpacker compared to a fully loaded RV. In other words, it uses fewer resources. When you choose plant-based meals over animal products, you're helping to lighten the load on our planet's resources. Think of it as doing more with less— less land, less water, less energy.

As mentioned, switching to a plant-based diet can significantly lower greenhouse gas emissions because it steers clear of animal agriculture, which, as we know, is a major emitter of methane and nitrous oxide. It's like swapping out a gas-guzzling vehicle for a sleek bicycle—you're still getting where you need to go but with a much smaller environmental footprint.

Water, our precious, life-giving resource, is also better preserved with a vegan diet. Plant-based meals typically require less water than those involving animal products. It's like fixing a leaky faucet in your house—it might not seem like much at first, but over time, you're saving a ton of water.

By going vegan, you're also helping the trees—and not simply in a metaphorical, hug-a-tree kind of way. Vegan diets help reduce the need for land clearance, which in turn supports forest preservation. This is crucial for keeping our air clean, our water cycles functioning, and our wildlife thriving. It's like being a guardian for the lungs of our planet.

Last but not least, a plant-based diet is a win for biodiversity. When we reduce the demand for animal products, we also reduce the pressure on ecosystems and habitats. This means more space for wildlife, more diverse plant life, and healthier ecosystems. It's giving nature a break so it can flourish in all its wonderful diversity.

Going vegan isn't only about the food on your plate; it's making choices that ripple outward to create a healthier, more sustainable world. Every plant-based meal is a step toward a greener, kinder planet, and that's something to feel good about.

Incorporating Compassion and Understanding into Your Daily Life

When we talk about adding a bit more compassion and understanding to our everyday lives, we're talking about cultivating empathy. We're turning up the dial on our ability to connect with others on a deeper level. Let's break down what this means and how to do it.

Cultivating Empathy

Empathy is like having a superpower; it's the ability to understand what someone else is feeling, to walk a mile in their shoes, so to speak. When you flex your empathy muscle, you're opening your heart a bit wider, making room for more kindness and deeper connections with the people in your life.

Now, here's a golden rule: listen more, judge less. When someone's talking to you, really tune in. I mean, put away the phone, forget about your grocery list, and listen. Ask questions that show you're genuinely interested in understanding their point of view. It's about creating a safe space where the other person feels heard and valued, without the fear of being judged.

Imagine slipping into someone else's shoes for a moment. How do their challenges feel from their perspective? What might their day-to-day life be like? This isn't merely about sympathy; it's about truly trying to grasp someone else's experience and emotions. It can be eye-opening and can change the way you respond to them.

You might not agree with everyone on everything, and that's fine. But there's often common ground to be found, some shared slice of life, be it as small as liking the same type of music or as big as shared life experiences. Finding that commonality can bridge gaps and foster empathy, even amidst differing opinions.

By weaving these threads of empathy into the fabric of your daily life, you're not only making your world a better place, but you're also contributing to a kinder, more compassionate world. It's about understanding that everyone has their own story, their own struggles and joys, and that understanding can be the first step toward a more empathetic, connected society.

Show Empathy Toward Animals

Showing empathy can extend beyond our fellow humans and companion animals. All furry, feathered, and finned species deserve compassion and understanding. They might not speak our language, but they have their own stories, feelings, and experiences.

First up, it's key to understand that animals are not simply creatures moving about on autopilot. They're sentient beings, meaning they can feel pain, joy, fear, and love, just like us. Understanding this about animal welfare is a great first step. Beyond the cats and dogs that we share our homes with, most people don't know how animals behave—or, more accurately, how they behave naturally in their natural environments. We need to educate ourselves about how animals live, what they need, and the challenges they face—especially those in factory farms or in captivity. This knowledge can be a real eye-opener, the foundation of genuine empathy, and a deep understanding of the horrific lives they face at the hands of humans.

One of the best ways to connect with animals and understand them better? Get involved! Volunteering at an animal shelter or sanctuary can be an incredible experience. You get to meet animals up close, understand their personalities and stories, and help make their lives better. It's like stepping into their world and seeing things from their point of view. If you're more into wildlife, observing animals in their natural habitat can be super insightful. Watching how they interact in the wild, in their own element, can give you a deeper appreciation for their instincts, behaviors, and the roles they play in the ecosystem.

Wouldn't you agree that it's a much better experience for humans to view them in their natural habitats? Go whale watching instead of supporting aquariums that think it's acceptable to capture, imprison, and train orcas and belugas and make them do tricks. Or invest in an adventure of a lifetime by seeing lions, cheetahs, giraffes, zebras, and countless other wildlife on a safari in Africa as opposed to behind bars in a zoo.

By developing this stronger understanding and empathy for animals, we start to see them in a new light. They're not here as background characters in our lives; they're living, feeling beings with their own place in the world. This shift in perspective can deeply enrich our lives, bringing a greater sense of connection to the natural world and all its inhabitants.

Make Kind Choices

The choices we make every day, big or small, can be a powerful form of kindness, especially when it comes to the products we use. We need to learn to make conscious decisions with our consumer dollars that reflect our compassion for animals and our stand against their mistreatment.

Each product you choose is casting a vote. When you opt for cruelty-free and vegan products, you're voting for a kinder world. These products are created without any animal testing and without any animal-derived ingredients. It's saying no to a process that causes harm and yes to a more ethical, compassionate approach.

Making the switch to cruelty-free and vegan products is making a statement. It's telling companies and industries that you care about how products are made, and that animal welfare matters to you. Every cruelty-free lotion, every vegan lipstick, and every animal-friendly cleaning product you purchase sends a message that kindness and compassion are priorities in your life.

By choosing these kinds of products, you're helping to decrease the demand for items that involve animal mistreatment. It's like pulling one small brick out of a large wall—with enough people doing it, eventually, the whole structure begins to wobble. Your choices no longer support unethical companies whose only concerns are for the bottom line; instead, you contribute to a growing movement that advocates for the ethical treatment of animals, not in words but in actions.

Making kind choices in our daily lives might seem like a small thing, but it's these little decisions that add up to create big changes. We need to be conscious of our impact and choose a path that aligns with our values. The next time you're out shopping, remember that each product you pick can be a reflection of your compassion and a step toward a more humane world. Remember, the road to veganism is a process—one item, one meal, one conscious, heartfelt decision in alignment with your compassion at a time.

Sharing the Message: Advocating and Educating

If you're passionate about veganism and want to share it with the world, I'm truly grateful. Let's talk about how you can spread the word effectively and, as importantly, kindly. It's about the art of communication and a dash of diplomacy.

Effective Communication

When it comes to advocating for veganism, it's not only what you say, but also how you say it. Picture yourself as a friendly guide, not a forceful debater. The goal is to have open, productive discussions where you share ideas and perspectives while sharing facts. You want to plant seeds and inspire people to ask questions and continue the conversation rather than shut down or argue.

Be aware that not everyone will be on the same page as you, and that's okay. When faced with criticism or skepticism, remember to keep your cool. Respond with understanding and patience.

Show grace under fire. When you handle criticism well, you're not simply defending veganism; you're embodying its compassionate spirit.

Advocate for veganism with the same kindness that's at the heart of the lifestyle. Judging or shaming others for their choices never works. Instead, inspire change through example, and share information in a way that's inviting, not alienating. Think of it as being a friendly source of information, rather than a pushy salesperson.

By developing these communication skills, you become an effective ambassador for veganism. You're speaking for a cause, opening a meaningful dialogue, and possibly leading others toward a more compassionate lifestyle. Remember, it's not about winning an argument; it's about winning hearts and minds, one kind conversation at a time.

Educating and Spreading Veganism

There are some creative ways to educate and spread the good word about veganism—a way of bringing the message to life. There are so many fun, engaging, and effective methods to get people curious and excited about this lifestyle.

Imagine throwing a vegan cooking class or a workshop on sustainable living. These events can be a fantastic way to bring people together, share experiences, and learn something new in a relaxed and friendly environment. It's like hosting a party where everyone leaves a bit more informed and inspired.

In this digital age, the world is your oyster when it comes to spreading ideas. Utilizing social media, blogs, or starting a YouTube channel can amplify your message far and wide. Share recipes, tips, personal stories, or the latest vegan or animal advocacy news. Create a space online where people can discover and explore veganism at their own pace.

Teaming up with local groups can help broaden your reach. Whether it's a community garden, a school, or a health fair, these collaborations can provide a platform for educating others about veganism and its benefits. Consider joining forces with other like-minded people to create a bigger, more impactful wave of change.

Think about designing programs or seminars that dive into various aspects of veganism—from health benefits to environmental impacts, and even ethical considerations. These can be held in schools, libraries, or community centers and are a great way to engage with people of all ages and backgrounds.

By embracing these diverse methods, you're bringing veganism into people's lives in tangible, accessible ways. Meet people where they are and invite them into a world of compassionate and sustainable living. Every workshop, post, collaboration, and program can be a stepping-stone for someone on their journey toward veganism.

Leading through Example

I touched on this already, but one of the most powerful ways to spread the vegan message is leading by example. You become a walking, talking billboard for the benefits of veganism, but in a cool, relatable way. Here's how you can be a role model and inspire others simply by being you.

Imagine your life as a showcase of what vegan living can do. When you're rocking a healthy, vibrant lifestyle, people can't help but notice.

You're an example of how nourishing and fulfilling a plant-based life can be. You don't even have to say much; your energy and health speak volumes.

As mentioned, being vegan is about more than food; it's a compassionate way of life. Showcasing kindness not only toward animals but also toward people can make a huge impact. It's like being a beacon of positivity and empathy. When folks see how compassion drives your choices and interactions, it can inspire them to think about their own.

By embodying this lifestyle, you create ripples that can extend far beyond your immediate circle. People get curious, they start asking questions, and before you know it, you're having meaningful conversations about veganism over coffee or at the gym. It's about igniting that spark of curiosity and leading by example.

Being a role model in veganism isn't about being perfect; it's about being genuine and approachable. It's showing the world that a vegan lifestyle is attainable, enjoyable, and rewarding. So, keep doing what you're doing, share your experiences, and let your life be the inspiration that could nudge someone else toward making compassionate choices. Who knows? Your example could be the catalyst for change in someone's life.

Collaborating for a Better Future

As I mentioned in a previous section, joining forces for the greater good is a great option. Going vegan is awesome, but imagine what we can achieve when we band together!

We've all heard the saying, "There's strength in numbers." That rings especially true in the world of vegan activism. Joining vegan groups or communities can supercharge your efforts. It's about pooling resources, sharing ideas, and supporting each other. Whether it's local meetups, online forums, or large organizations, there's a whole world of collective action you can tap into.

Get involved in community events, sign petitions, bear witness, join peaceful demonstrations—every bit counts. Each of us is a puzzle piece, and when we come together, we create a powerful picture of change and advocacy.

Beyond individual actions, think about the bigger picture. Supporting policy changes, advocating for animal rights, and promoting sustainable practices can make waves in society. Use your voice and your vote to influence larger societal and environmental shifts.

We've explored the ethical heart of veganism, dived into its environmental impact, busted some myths, and talked about how to spread the word effectively. But most importantly, I've shared how veganism is more than a diet; it's a way of life grounded in compassion and sustainability.

This chapter is a call to action, inviting you to be part of a compassionate and eco-friendly future. It's a reminder that your choices, your voice, and your actions matter. Whether you're a new or seasoned vegan, remember that every step you take toward a more compassionate and sustainable lifestyle is a step in the right direction.

I encourage you to keep learning, advocating, and making those kind choices. Together, we can make a difference for the animals, our planet, and ourselves. Here's to moving forward with compassion and determination, one plant-based choice at a time.

CHAPTER 7

Your Holistic Wellness Adventure

This chapter provides insights into the exciting world of holistic wellness. Think of it as your all-in-one self-care package, a toolkit for nurturing your body, mind, and spirit. I share what I have discovered to be the best elements to create a life that's not only balanced but also deeply fulfilling.

In the pages ahead, you're going to discover how to seamlessly blend practices like yoga, meditation, mindfulness, and regular exercise into your daily routine. We're moving beyond the occasional stretch or moment of silence. This is about crafting a lifestyle that brings out the best in you across the board.

For those who have never practiced yoga, I provide a basic framework for understanding that it's not about contorting into complex shapes but rather finding balance and harmony. Meditation then steps in as your secret weapon for mental clarity and calmness. A few minutes each day can be a game-changer.

Think of mindfulness as your daily dose of clarity and presence. Whether sipping morning coffee or commuting, it invites us to fully immerse ourselves in these moments.

With exercise, I'm going to share my view that it can be genuinely fun and uplifting. From a heart-pumping dance session to a refreshing stroll in your local park where you can enjoy nature and wildlife, it's a matter of choosing movement that makes you feel most alive.

As we explore these practices, our focus is on making them both practical and enjoyable. No matter where you are on your wellness path, I encourage you to use this guide as a starting point for inspiration. Let's dive in and embrace wellness as an enriching, enjoyable journey!

Yoga: Uniting Body and Mind

Yoga is an ancient practice that transcends time and place, but its benefits are as relevant today as they were centuries ago. It's not simply a form of physical exercise; it's a journey of self-discovery and a powerful tool for enhancing physical health and mental clarity. As you explore different yoga poses, each breath and movement deepen your connection with yourself.

Yoga teaches us about patience, resilience, and self-compassion. With each session, you may find yourself becoming more flexible in both body and mind. Remember, yoga is a holistic practice encompassing mental and spiritual aspects, bringing peace and clarity to your busy life.

Every time you step onto your mat is an opportunity to strengthen, calm, and balance yourself. Yoga harmonizes your physical health with your mental and emotional well-being, paving the way for a more balanced and fulfilling life.

There are multiple styles of yoga, each with its unique flavor. Whether it's the steady pace of Hatha, the dynamic flow of Vinyasa, the discipline of Ashtanga, the precision of Iyengar, the intensity of Bikram/Hot Yoga, the spiritual depth of Kundalini, the soothing touch of Restorative Yoga, or the meditative focus of Yin Yoga, there's a style that resonates with every soul. Experiment, try out different classes, and find the style that speaks to your needs. Your perfect yoga journey awaits!

Mindful Movement in Yoga

Yoga is also a form of moving meditation. By synchronizing your movement with your breath and savoring every sensation, you turn each session into a mindful experience. You learn to move with intention, stay present with your thoughts, and find moments of tranquility between poses. This mindful approach to yoga enriches your practice, marrying the physical with the mental for a holistic experience.

Every Body Can Practice Yoga

Yoga truly is for everyone; regardless of your age, level of flexibility, body shape, or stage in life, there's a spot on the yoga mat for you. From local studios and gyms to online platforms and community centers, the perfect yoga class is out there. Embrace props and modifications, connect with the yoga community, and find the class that fits your journey.

Your Mental Reset Button

Meditation is like hitting the pause button in a fast-paced life. Starting with a few minutes a day in a quiet corner, you can explore different meditation styles—guided, silent, or mantra-based. Explore and try the different styles to discover what resonates with you and embrace the learning curve. You may want to practice all forms, depending on how you feel on any given day. Regular meditation can lead to greater peace, clarity, and mindfulness, making it a precious part of your daily routine.

The Art of Being Present

Mindfulness transforms ordinary tasks into extraordinary moments of joy and discovery. Practice being fully present in simple daily activities, whether it's enjoying a meal, doing the dishes, or going for a walk. Engage in mindful conversations, listening actively and deeply to others. This practice opens a window to more authentic interactions and a deeper connection with the present moment. By embracing mindfulness, you step off the autopilot mode of life, taking control of the steering wheel to fully experience and savor each moment. Remember, in these instances of mindfulness, life's colors shine their brightest.

Finding Joy in Movement

Redefine exercise as a source of joy, not a chore. Identify activities that ignite your enthusiasm and make you feel alive. Consider dancing to your favorite tunes, exploring nature on a hike, or taking a rejuvenating swim; choose activities that you genuinely enjoy so that you will look forward to doing them and you will be consistent. Listen to your body's cues—it tells you what it needs, whether it's an energetic workout or a gentler activity. This approach transforms exercise from a routine task into a celebration of your body's capabilities and a way to elevate your mood and well-being.

Creating Your Wellness Plan

Your wellness journey is as unique as you are, and your plan should reflect that individuality. Mix and match practices like yoga, meditation, cardiovascular conditioning, weight-bearing exercise, and mindfulness in a way that fits your lifestyle. Be flexible and open to adapting your plan as your needs evolve. This isn't about rigid routines; it's about crafting a living, evolving practice that supports your well-being and brings joy to your daily life. Embrace the process of creating and adjusting your wellness plan; it's your personal blueprint for a healthier, happier you.

Here's a sample week to inspire your wellness journey:

- Monday: Start with a morning meditation, choose a midday walk for a dose of vitamin D, and then end your day with an evening yoga session.
- Tuesday: Set your intentions with morning journaling, enjoy a healthy lunch, and engage in evening strength training.
- Wednesday: Greet the day with gentle stretching, take a nature walk at lunch, and unwind with a guided meditation at night.
- Thursday: Begin with a gratitude practice, stretch during your lunch

break, and enjoy a fun dance class in the evening.

- Friday: Energize with morning breathwork, try a relaxing afternoon stroll, and socialize or relax in the evening.
- Saturday: Indulge in a longer yoga practice or a meditation session, try a new outdoor activity, and enjoy a self-care evening routine.
- Sunday: Take a leisurely walk mid-morning while reflecting on your week, focus on nutritious meal prep for the week ahead in the afternoon, and spend some time in the evening setting goals for the coming week.

Navigating Life's Ups and Downs

Life's roller-coaster brings challenges, but they are chances for growth and learning. Treat yourself with kindness and understanding during tough times, like you would a dear friend. Lean on your community for support, whether it's sharing after a yoga class or having meaningful conversations with friends and like-minded people. Consider what I've shared as your companion on a journey of self-discovery and holistic wellness, offering steps toward a more balanced, joyful, and fulfilling life. Embrace the journey and remember—you're doing an incredible job on this path of growth and well-being.

Evolving and Thriving with a Plant-Based Lifestyle

Get ready to dive deep into the thrilling journey of growth and development that accompanies adopting a plant-based lifestyle. As your faithful guide, I will share my experiences and emphasize the significance of embracing change and constantly learning.

My journey toward adopting a plant-based lifestyle is not unique, however, my convictions and actions have evolved over the years.

Personal Growth and Self-Discovery

My path to a plant-based lifestyle started with self-reflection and introspection. My upbringing, cultural background, health concerns, and moral principles influenced my decision to explore plant-based living. Through studying, trial and error, and education, I gradually transitioned to a plant-based way of life. It's about keeping an open mind and constantly evolving our beliefs and behaviors.

Throughout my journey, there were pivotal moments that solidified my dedication to a plant-based lifestyle. These moments include trying new and exciting foods, attending vegan gatherings, and building connections with individuals who share my beliefs. Through these experiences, I recognized the incredible benefits of living a plant-based life, not only for myself but also for the environment and other living creatures.

As I embraced a plant-based lifestyle, I incorporated its values into all aspects of my life. This meant choosing sustainable fashion options, minimizing waste, and advocating for animal rights. Through this journey, my empathy, compassion, and mindfulness have expanded and I'm always striving for personal growth. As Maya Angelou once said, "When you know better, you do better." I believe in embracing the process of continuous improvement without pressuring oneself to conform to a certain way of living.

In short, my ceaseless exploration of the plant-based lifestyle serves as motivation for those seeking to make similar changes in their own lives. It highlights the impact of self-discovery, growth, and aligning our beliefs with our behaviors. I encourage you to embrace change and continue progressing on your path toward overall well-being.

There may be challenges when transitioning to a plant-based diet, but there are ways to overcome those obstacles. And along the way, it's important to celebrate your successes in your quest for optimal health and wellness.

Transitioning to a plant-based lifestyle means changing habits that have been ingrained since childhood and can also include facing criticism from society. This is when I leaned on self-reflection, determination, and support from loved ones to help me deal with these challenges while remaining true to my reasons for choosing to eliminate animal products from my life.

When you face your challenges head-on, you emerge stronger and wiser. I gained a deeper understanding of the value of patience, resilience, and adaptability when facing obstacles. Additionally, I uncovered innovative techniques for preparing food and planning meals that improved my overall well-being.

In the midst of facing obstacles, I always made sure to take time to recognize any small victories. Whether it was perfecting a delicious new dish or hitting a fitness goal, acknowledging these achievements served as fuel for my determination to reach bigger objectives.

Living a vegan lifestyle deeply impacted my perspective on existence. It revealed to me the interdependence of all living creatures and our planet. This change motivated me to adopt a more conscious mindset toward food decisions and consumption, promoting not only my health but also the well-being of the world.

While transitioning to a plant-based lifestyle can be challenging, the benefits are significant. It highlights the value of perseverance, gaining knowledge from obstacles, and acknowledging accomplishments throughout the process. No difficulty is too great to conquer on this journey, and personal growth and development are achievable through embracing change.

Life is an ever-flowing river of change, like the changing of seasons. Like nature, our lives are constantly evolving. Instead of resisting change with fear and resistance, approach it with curiosity and openness.

When faced with setbacks in areas such as health, relationships, or careers, it can be overwhelming. But we can all learn to adapt to unfamiliar situations and gracefully navigate them. Being open-minded and adaptable are crucial factors in successfully overcoming these obstacles.

Welcoming New Opportunities

When we welcome change, we unlock new doors of potential and chances for personal development. Let go of restrictive thoughts and embrace different points of view; this goes a long way toward promoting change, leading to more enriching experiences in life.

As we continue to grow and change, our bodies and needs do as well, so it's important to be flexible in your personal growth journeys. This entails experimenting with different methods and regularly evaluating what is most effective for you.

Discovering the Advantages of Embracing Change

Opening ourselves up to change offers valuable lessons. We become improved iterations of who we are by pushing past our comfort zones, facing obstacles head-on, and adjusting accordingly.

We all need to learn to accept change because it's part of life and not something to be afraid of. By embracing change and remaining adaptable on your unique path, you can flourish. Explore the constantly changing world of the plant-based movement and find ways to remain up-to-date and flexible.

Remaining Knowledgeable

The world of veganism and plant-based living is ever-evolving. Become empowered by staying informed so you can easily make the best decisions and choices for your well-being and lifestyle, from the latest research findings to emerging trends.

Making Changes to Eating Habits

As you learn more about the benefits of a plant-based diet, your eating habits may need to evolve. For optimum health, focus on whole foods and minimizing processed options. It's a trap many new to plant-based eating fall into—packaged and processed foods, but these plant-based versions are no healthier than their animal-based counterparts.

Try integrating new insights into your existing routines rather than completely overhauling everything at once. This balanced approach to incorporating new information allows for sustainable adjustments and avoids overwhelming pressure.

Differentiating Between Sustainable Practices

In any movement, there are always fleeting trends. Remember to recognize the difference between sustainable practices and passing fads.

Instead of turning to temporary fixes and extreme diets, prioritize long-term health and wellness.

Being curious and open-minded is essential when navigating the ever-changing landscape of plant-based living. I can't stress enough the value of continuous learning and experimentation in finding your unique approach to a plant-based lifestyle. Stay informed, adaptable, and mindful as you navigate the constantly evolving world of plant-based living. By staying open to new information and incorporating it into your daily routines when appropriate, you can continue making strides toward achieving a plant-based lifestyle.

There's tremendous value in continuously learning and striving for self-improvement in every aspect of our lives; they are essential components for our personal growth. Consider growth as a lifelong journey, rather than a final goal to reach, and it's important for every aspect of our lives—emotional, mental, spiritual, as well as physical well-being. These elements are all essential for our development as individuals.

Invaluable Resources

At the back of the book, I've provided a variety of resources, ranging from literature on nutrition and wellness to engaging podcasts and informative documentaries about plant-based lifestyles. These valuable resources can enhance your understanding and knowledge.

My strategies for achieving a balanced and fulfilling life while striving for self-improvement include setting goals, expressing gratitude, being present in the moment, finding a healthy work-life balance, and regularly evaluating and adjusting priorities.

Please know that self-discovery and growth are ongoing processes. Adopting a plant-based lifestyle is a holistic approach to living. Personal development is a journey filled with challenges and triumphs. Stay curious, open-minded, and dedicated to your path of self-improvement.

CHAPTER 9

Developing a Strong Support System

There is strength in the community formed when embracing a plant-based lifestyle. Community is a powerful influence on adopting and sustaining this way of living, so it's worth spending some time exploring some of the strategies we can use to help us connect with others who share our values and beliefs, both online and offline. This not only enhances our personal journey but also contributes to the advancement of the plant-based movement as a whole.

Establishing a Supportive Network

A great way to build relationships with individuals who share similar beliefs is by joining online communities and physical locations that foster plant-based communities.

I discovered a community through online groups and local gatherings, and I can't stress enough the significance of forming connections with like-minded individuals who hold similar principles and convictions.

Here are some potential steps to help you get involved.

Online Platforms

In this digital age, it is easier than ever to connect with like-minded individuals all over the world. Social media platforms, forums, and virtual groups provide opportunities to share experiences, exchange ideas, and receive support.

Seek guidance and support through reputable online sources that align with your values and beliefs.

Getting Involved

Active participation in conversations and events within these communities is essential for building relationships and developing a strong support system.

Communicate about plant-based values and beliefs with openness, respect, and empathy.

Push past your comfort zone and attend events or join activities in person where you can meet and connect with like-minded individuals.

Participate in Meaningful Discussions

Being an active member of these communities means engaging in conversations and events. It's not enough to just be present; it's important to actively contribute.

Communicate the values and beliefs of a plant-based lifestyle with openness, respect, and empathy.

Also, try seeking out events and activities where like-minded individuals can connect and share their plant-based journeys. Stepping out of one's comfort zone can lead to valuable relationships and connections.

Benefits of Having a Community

Being a member of a supportive community has many advantages for those who choose to live a plant-based lifestyle.

Let's explore these advantages:

- Sense of belonging: A community provides a sense of belonging, which can be especially valuable for those on a less conventional dietary journey.

- Encouragement and support: Like-minded individuals in the community offer moral support and motivation, helping to maintain one's commitment to plant-based values.

- Opportunities for learning: Communities are valuable sources of knowledge. You can learn from others' experiences, discover new recipes, and share meal ideas.

- Building relationships: Connecting with others who share your values and interests can be deeply fulfilling and create strong bonds within the community.

- Making an impact: Your participation in the community contributes to the growth and acceptance of the plant-based movement, making a positive impact on a larger scale.

Be intentional about connecting with others who share similar beliefs to build a network of support on your path. Actively seek out like-minded individuals and build meaningful relationships that can enhance your journey. Joining a larger community not only offers emotional support, but also provides chances for personal growth, learning, and making a positive impact in the plant-based movement. By forming these connections, we have the power to create real change for ourselves, our community, and the world.

CHAPTER 10

Moving Forward

This last step on your path toward adopting a plant-based lifestyle is like a motivational speech from your coach after completing a marathon. It's a time to look back, acknowledge your accomplishments, and plan for the future ahead.

Pausing to Reflect on the Journey So Far

Inhale deeply and take a moment to appreciate how much progress you've made. I've shared what I know and the lessons I've learned from my own journey, complete with some bumps in the road.

My health transformation has been eye-opening. I now have more energy, glowing skin, and a well-functioning digestive system. By tuning into my body's needs and prioritizing self-care, I have achieved these results. And you can too!

This transformation is not only evident in my physical health. My mindset has undergone a complete makeover. For me, food is now more than a source of energy; it's also a means of nourishment and happiness. I have developed a newfound appreciation for food and a healthier approach to eating.

Throughout my journey, there have been moments of intense cravings, and I found ways to overcome them, including practicing mindfulness and opting for plant-based and vegan options to satisfy my cravings. At this stage in my life, I no longer experience cravings. Instead, I have steadfast determination, and despite the obstacles, I remain focused on thriving on a plant-based lifestyle. This determination has also had a positive impact on other facets of my life, making me an unstoppable force.

Taking time to reflect on your journey is like consulting a compass; it provides direction and insight into how much progress has been made. It serves as a reminder of the initial motivation behind embarking on this endeavor, not only for physical well-being but also for personal development.

The plant-based community is a powerful force in the world of food and health. It has grown significantly over time, thanks to increased attention on animal welfare, environmental awareness, and its health benefits. Organizations such as The Vegetarian Society and The Vegan Society have laid the groundwork for this movement, providing resources for those looking to adopt a plant-based lifestyle.

In recent years, the popularity of plant-based diets has skyrocketed, with new vegan food companies, restaurants offering vegan options, and an increasing number of people participating in initiatives like Veganuary. But perhaps the most valuable aspect of this community is the support system it provides. With online forums, local meetups, cookbooks, and blogs dedicated to plant-based living, it's like being part of a tight-knit family that understands and supports your choices. This sense of community can be likened to having a coach on your team, boosting your confidence, offering guidance, and reminding you that you are not alone in your journey toward a healthier, more compassionate lifestyle. It's a tribe of like-minded individuals who have each other's back.

The growth within the plant-based community should be celebrated. Businesses are now offering more plant-based options, vegan athletes are breaking records and gaining recognition, and influencers are increasing awareness about living an animal-free lifestyle. It's important to recognize and give credit to the entire community for their efforts in promoting progress and change.

It feels like a celebration of all the hard work being done to create a kinder, more environmentally friendly world. Every small step is significant, and the community is making incredible progress.

Looking Ahead: The Evolution of a Holistic and Plant-Based Lifestyle

Let's turn our gaze toward the future—your future in a world focused on plant-based living.

Technology is becoming your partner in this journey, making it easier and more convenient to choose plant-based options. Imagine a world where tasty and realistic alternatives to animal products are the norm.

Sustainability is key. Your food choices play a crucial role in creating a greener and more sustainable environment. As awareness grows, farming practices will shift toward an eco-friendlier approach.

Inclusion is on the horizon. Every person should have access to plant-based choices, regardless of their location or income. You are part of a movement that advocates for equal access to healthy and sustainable food options.

As a bonus, there is holistic living. It goes beyond what you eat—it's about mindfulness, self-care, and making sustainable choices. It shows that you care about yourself, the planet, and all living beings.

Vision for the Future: A Continuous Journey of Development and Discovery

This is not an ending, but the beginning of something even more incredible. Adopting a plant-based lifestyle is not a destination; it's a dynamic process of education and evolution.

As your guide in this book, I want to remind you that this journey is unique to you. It's about making choices that align with your values, health goals, and daily life. Don't let obstacles discourage you or derail your efforts; instead, use them as opportunities to learn. Keep an open mind and stay curious.

Take Action: Join the Movement

Stay connected and become part of the plant-based community, whether online, locally, or globally.

Spread the message, whether that's through sharing your story or what you've learned along the way. Your journey contributes to the growing movement of plant-based living and its positive impact.

Remember these important lessons:

1. There are advantages to your health for following a plant-based lifestyle. Learn about the nutritional benefits, spot and dispel common misconceptions, and enjoy

exploring the delicious world of plant-based cuisine.

2. View this as a holistic approach to wellness. Health is not only about what you eat; it's also about mindfulness, physical activity, and overall well-being.

3. Keep the ethical and environmental considerations for transitioning to a vegan lifestyle top of mind. Become aware of the impact your choices have on animals and the planet.

4. Get involved in building a community and advocating for change. This community provides many opportunities to connect with others who share your passion for living a plant-based life and to spread awareness about its benefits.

5. There's always more to learn, both formally and informally. There's no lack of free information and valid research on all the benefits of a vegan world. And if it calls to you, consider formal training, such as the Plant-Based Nutrition Certification through the Center for Nutrition Studies. Continue to grow and learn in whatever way suits your budget and available time.

It's important for all of us to keep evolving as we continue this journey. It's all part of the process.

I hope you consider this the beginning of a new chapter. Your venture into the world of plant-based living is an ongoing tale of self-discovery and expansion. The resources I provided are merely the tip of the iceberg in terms of what's available for you, and much of it for free.

I'm always here to support you in your ongoing exploration of this nourishing, holistic lifestyle.

I'm rooting for you and reminding you that this journey is yours alone. Keep making choices that align with your values and well-being. Remember, challenges are simply stepping-stones on the path to success. Stay open-minded, be kind to yourself, and continue moving forward with determination.

Building on Your Plant-Based Journey: Additional Resources and Next Steps

Please be sure to review all the resources I've listed in the Appendices. You'll find listings for books, podcasts, documentaries, social media accounts, websites, cookbooks, and apps.

Books, Podcasts, Documentaries, Cookbooks, Apps, and Online Resources

Here are additional resources to support your continued exploration of a plant-based lifestyle. Remember, this is not only about what you eat; it's about transforming your entire being and making a positive impact on the world. Every small change can lead to a ripple effect beyond your own life. Thank you for joining me on this adventure, and may your path toward holistic, plant-based living continue to flourish and develop.

Recommended Books:

The China Study by T. Colin Campbell. This well-researched book reveals the amazing health benefits of a plant-based diet through solid scientific evidence.

How Not to Die by Dr. Michael Greger is a comprehensive guide to preventing and reversing chronic diseases by making lifestyle choices.

Eating Animals by Jonathan Safran Foer. This book offers a heartfelt discussion about the ethical implications of our food choices.

Byron Katie's *Loving What Is* is a guide that will take you through the powerful method she has developed using real-life examples. This book will teach you how to use this groundbreaking process for yourself, in a clear and easy-to-follow manner.

The Mindful Vegan by Lani Muelrath: Explore the intersection of mindfulness, plant-based living, and self-improvement.

Jumpstart Your Life by Diane Randall, M.A.: Learn how to use discomfort as a catalyst for personal development and change.

In his book *The Myth of Normal*, Gabor Maté examines the increasing prevalence of chronic illness and overall poor health in Western countries, despite their supposed excellent healthcare systems.

The Joyful Vegan: How to Stay Vegan in a World That Wants You to Eat Meat, Dairy, and Eggs, by Colleen Patrick-Goudreau. Master communicator,

Colleen provides strategies for talking with loved ones about your choice to become vegan, and she offers solutions to some common challenges.

Authors and registered dietitians Brenda Davis and Vesanto Melina team up with agrologist Cory Davis in their book *Plant-Powered Protein* to expose the misconceptions and political influences surrounding plant-based protein.

Online resources to help with a transition to veganism include:

Plant Based Curious: Delve into the world of plant-based nutrition, holistic living, veganism, and transforming behavior.

Food for Thought, with Colleen Patrick-Goudreau. This podcast program has been produced for decades. It's considered the leading resource for "living compassionately and healthfully" and Patrick-Goudreau has a gift for language and clarifying complex subjects.

The Vegan Fitness Podcast, with Fritz Horstmann.

Nutrition Facts with Dr. Greger.

The Happy Pear with twin brothers Steve and Dave Flynn in Ireland.

No Meat Athlete Radio with Matt Fraser.

On Instagram, you'll get lots of recipe ideas from @broccoli_mum, @plantyou, @start_veganmeal, @maxlamanna, @_spicymoustache_, @schoolnightvegan, @dereksarno, @plantbasedonabudget, @thekoreanvegan, and @fitgreenmind.

On YouTube, you can't go wrong with Jane Esselstyn and Ann Crile Esselstyn, daughter and wife of Caldwell B. Esselstyn, Jr., M.D. respectively. Find them at @JaneEsselstyn.

Also on YouTube, you can find Miyoko Schinner @thevegangoodlifewithmiyoko.

NutritionFacts.org: Keep up to date on the latest nutritional research through easily accessible videos.

VeganSociety.com offers guidance and resources on all aspects of veganism, including nutrition, health, environmental impact, and animal rights.

PlantBasedNews.org: Explore articles and join a community focused on veganism and eco-friendly living.

DianeRandallConsults.com: Utilize valuable resources to create the life you have always dreamed of.

WeDidIt.Health has excellent expert interviews, which you can access via their YouTube channel: youtube.com/@wedidit.health. Subscribe to the channel for regular updates.

Visual Learning through Documentaries

Sometimes, seeing is believing. These documentaries offer in-depth perspectives on plant-based living:

Forks Over Knives: An exploration into the link between animal products and chronic diseases.

Cowspiracy: A shocking revelation about the environmental impact of animal agriculture.

You Are What You Eat: Investigating the connection between diet and disease in American twins.

Dominion: Exposes the dark side of modern animal agriculture and raises questions about the morality and validity of humankind's dominion over the animal kingdom.

Fuel Your Culinary Creativity with Cookbooks

Embark on a delicious adventure in plant-based cooking. Expand your skills and add new flavors to your journey with the help of cookbooks. Here are a few of my top suggestions.

Oh She Glows, by Angela Liddon.

The Prevent and Reverse Heart Disease Cookbook, by Ann Crile Esselstyne and Jane Esselstyn.

PlantYou and *PlantYou Scrappy Cooking* by Carleigh Bodrug. Carleigh is at the @PlantYou handle on Instagram I mentioned above where she has more than five million followers.

The PlantPure Nation Cookbook by Kim Campbell.

Forks Over Knives, The Cookbook, by Del Sroufe.

Here are three mobile apps that can help enhance your well-being:

Yuka: By scanning barcodes, this app provides useful insights into the nutritional value of products, making it simpler to select healthier options.

Ingred: This app allows users to search its database for food additives and ingredients in cosmetics, highlighting those that may negatively impact one's health.

Happy Cow: This app makes finding and accessing healthy food more convenient and accessible.

Menu Samples and Recipes

To help you get started on your plant-based journey, here are a few menu options:

A Week in the Life of Someone New to Plant-Based Eating

Day 1:

Breakfast: Begin your day with a bowl of overnight oats topped with plump berries and creamy almond milk.

Lunch: Indulge in a nourishing quinoa salad filled with an assortment of vibrant veggies.

Dinner: Warm up with a filling bowl of lentil soup served alongside steamed broccoli.

Day 2:

Breakfast: Experience a flavorful tofu scramble with a mix of fresh spinach, ripe tomato, and creamy avocado served on hearty whole wheat toast.

Lunch: Satisfy your taste buds with a hummus wrap made with roasted vegetables and wrapped in a whole wheat tortilla.

Dinner: Treat yourself to a nutritious baked sweet potato topped with protein-packed black beans, zesty salsa, and rich avocado.

Day 3:

Breakfast: Start your day with a refreshing green smoothie made of spinach, banana, and almond milk.

Lunch: Try a chickpea salad sandwich on whole-grain bread.

Dinner: End your day with a flavorful vegetable stir-fry served over aromatic brown rice.

Day 4

Breakfast: Start your morning with the delicious combination of avocado and tomato on top of toast, drizzled with balsamic glaze.

Lunch: Indulge in a hearty bowl of lentil and vegetable soup, accompanied by whole-grain crackers.

Dinner: Savor grilled portobello mushrooms over a bed of quinoa and steamed vegetables as a healthy and tasty option.

Day 5

Breakfast: Delight in fluffy buckwheat pancakes topped with seasonal fruit and a touch of maple syrup.

Lunch: Indulge in a hearty spinach salad filled with chickpeas, roasted veggies, and tangy balsamic dressing.

Dinner: Enjoy a dish of spaghetti squash smothered in rich marinara sauce and surrounded by sautéed vegetables.

Day 6

Morning Meal: Energize yourself with a deliciously creamy mango smoothie bowl topped with crunchy granola, nuts, and seeds.

Midday Meal: Savor a satisfying lentil stew served on a bed of nutritious brown rice.

Evening Meal: Add some flavor to your day with homemade mushroom fajitas spiced just right and wrapped in whole wheat tortillas.

Day 7

Breakfast: Start your morning with a flavorful tofu scramble, packed with spinach and mushrooms, served on whole grain toast.

Lunch: Indulge in a satisfying chickpea avocado wrap paired with garlic-roasted Brussels sprouts.

Dinner: Relish in the delicious combination of quinoa-stuffed bell peppers and balsamic-glazed carrots.

Consider the following for snacks in between meals:

- Apple with a small handful of nuts
- Carrot sticks with hummus
- Crackers with natural peanut butter or almond butter

- Smoothie made with oat milk, fruit and a handful of spinach

Below are four delicious recipes to add to your plant-based menu.

Creamy Avocado Pasta
Serves 2 to 3

Ingredients:

- 150 grams dry whole-wheat pasta
- 1 ripe avocado, roughly chopped
- 2 cloves of garlic
- Juice from one lemon
- 1 cup of cherry tomatoes, halved
- Fresh basil to taste

Directions:

- Cook the pasta according to package directions.
- Blend the avocado, garlic, and lemon juice. Add water if needed for desired consistency. Once smooth, toss the pasta with the sauce.

- Top with cherry tomatoes and basil for added flavor.

Cauliflower Buffalo Wings

Ingredients:

- 1 small to medium cauliflower, broken into florets
- ½ cup of whole wheat flour
- 1 teaspoon each of garlic powder, onion powder, paprika, and cumin
- ¾ cup unsweetened plant milk
- Salt and pepper to taste
- Hot sauce

Directions:

- Preheat oven to 375°F.
- To make these tasty wings, mix the flour with the spices and plant milk, then coat the cauliflower pieces in this batter. Bake for 15 minutes, turning after 10 minutes.
- Remove from the oven and brush with hot sauce and bake for another 10 minutes for an extra kick.

Vegan Chili

This is a hearty vegan chili.

Ingredients:

- 1 can of kidney beans
- 1 can of black beans
- 1 can of diced tomatoes
- 1 bell pepper, green, yellow, or orange, diced
- 1 yellow onion, diced
- 1 can of corn kernels, or 1 cup of frozen corn
- Spices to taste:
  Chili powder
  Cumin
  Paprika

Directions:

- In a large pot or Dutch oven, sauté onions and bell peppers before adding chili powder, cumin, and paprika. Next, stir in kidney beans, black beans, diced tomatoes, and corn. Simmer for 30 minutes.

Lentil Shepherd's Pie:

Ingredients:

- 6 to 8 potatoes suitable for mashing
- 1½ cups of brown or green lentils
- 4 cups of vegetable broth
- 1 onion
- Mixed vegetables, such as corn, peas, and carrots (a 10-ounce bag of frozen mixed vegetables works well)
- 2 Tablespoons of tomato paste
- 1 tablespoon of maple syrup
- 1 tablespoon of balsamic vinegar

Directions:

- Preheat oven to 425°F. Prepare a 2-quart baking dish.
- Cook the potatoes and mash to your preference—plant milk, vegan butter, etc. Set aside.
- In a large saucepan over medium heat, sauté onion in a bit of oil (or water if oil-free) and cook until translucent.

- Add lentils and broth and cook until tender—about 35 to 40 minutes. In the last 10 minutes of cooking, add the vegetables. Once lentils are tender, remove the cover and simmer to evaporate any excess liquid, stirring frequently to prevent sticking.
- Layer the cooked lentils with mixed vegetables in a baking dish. Mix maple syrup, tomato paste, and vinegar then pour over the vegetable layer. Finally, top with the mashed potatoes and bake until golden and bubbly.

I hope these recipe suggestions help get your creative juices flowing in the kitchen. Everyone's journey is different; explore, experiment, access the resources I've provided, and, most of all, enjoy this new chapter of living a healthier, kinder life.

Notes

Notes

Notes

Notes

Notes

Notes

Notes

Notes

Notes

Notes

About the Author

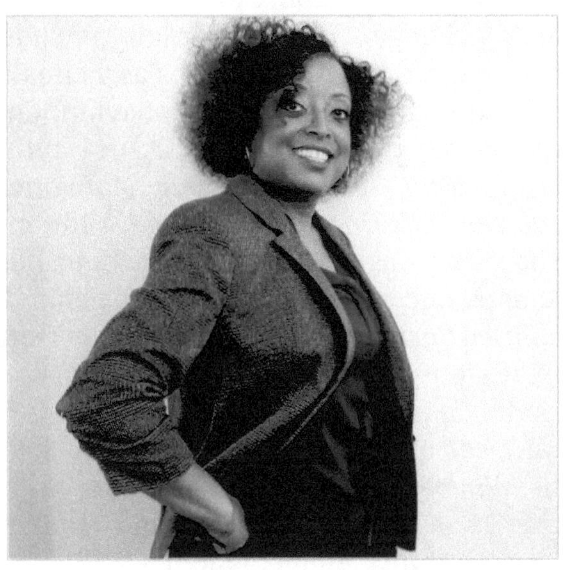

Join Diane Randall, M.A., CHC, on a transformative journey that will change your life. With over 20 years of experience as a whole living consultant, Diane is committed to helping busy professionals achieve overall well-being. She focuses on creating harmony, holistic wellness, promoting self-care, and embracing a plant-based lifestyle, empowering individuals to make healthy choices every day. Drawing from her personal experience living a plant-based and vegan lifestyle, Diane brings a wealth of knowledge to the world of wellness.

Utilizing her extensive knowledge and background in Spiritual Psychology, Diane provides valuable support to individuals seeking personal change. Her education includes a master's degree and certifications as a Life Coach, Holistic Health Coach, and Behavior Change Coach. Prior to this book, Diane authored *Jumpstart Your Life: Find Your Motivation to Change Your Life One Step at a Time*. Additionally, she shares her insights through teaching, hosting workshops, and engaging listeners on her podcast, *Plant Based Curious*. Her writing has been featured in prestigious publications like the *New York Times* and *Consulting Magazine*, and she has made appearances on prominent platforms such as the *Oprah Winfrey Show*. With over 30 years of experience as an SAP Consultant and Trainer, she has successfully implemented software for corporations both domestically and internationally while offering coaching services worldwide.

Are you ready to begin your journey toward wellness? Join Diane and her wealth of resources at www.dianerandallconsults.com. Discover a variety of tools such as books, workshops, group coaching sessions, podcasts, and more. Take the first step toward holistic well-being today.